An Introduction to CrossFit

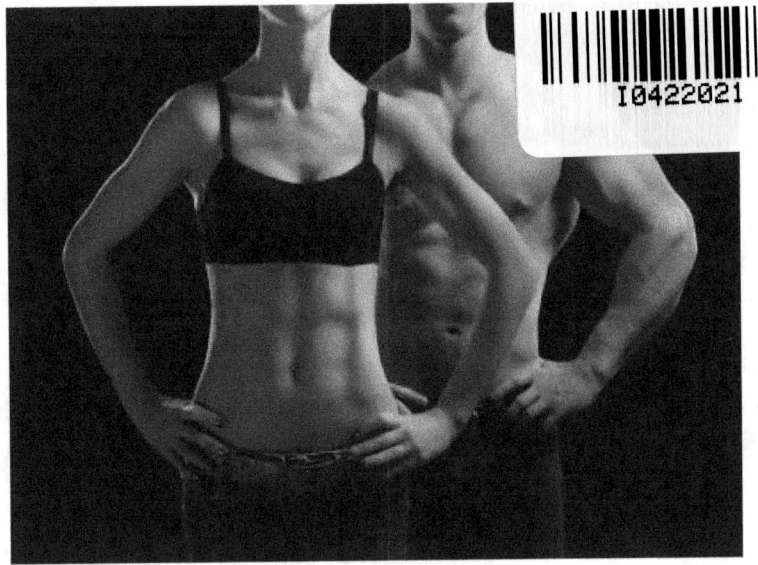

Health Learning Series

M. Usman

Mendon Cottage Books

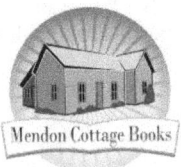

JD-Biz Publishing

Disclaimer

The information is this book is provided for informational purposes only. It is not intended to be used and medical advice or a substitute for proper medical treatment by a qualified health care provider. The information is believed to be accurate as presented based on research by the author.

The contents have not been evaluated by the U.S. Food and Drug Administration or any other Government or Health Organization and the contents in this book are not to be used to treat cure or prevent disease.

The author or publisher is not responsible for the use or safety of any diet, procedure or treatment mentioned in this book. The author or publisher is not responsible for errors or omissions that may exist.

Warning

The Book is for informational purposes only and before taking on any diet, treatment or medical procedure, it is recommended to consult with your primary health care provider.

Our books are available at

1. Amazon.com
2. Barnes and Noble
3. Itunes
4. Kobo
5. Smashwords
6. Google Play Books

Table of Contents

Preface

Having a great body that looks like a million dollar athlete or someone on a magazine cover, is a dream for many of us. It is usually accompanied with having lots of strength and being capable of doing just about anything that requires some muscle. Although, the unfortunate truth is that anyone who has ever tried this knows how difficult it is.

However, CrossFit might be a good answer to achieving this dream. Unlike bodybuilders who spend countless hours working a single muscle, CrossFit gets every muscle involved – even those you never thought you had. And since it can get lonely at the gym, CrossFit is more of a community. When in the box, there is so much motivation from friends that it is rare to see someone fail in achieving their goals.

CrossFit has helped people lose fat, become strong, and look great. It is basically strength and endurance training combined. This book will give you an introduction to what CrossFit is, how you can get started, and other related topics to help you reach your fitness goals.

So, read on!

Introduction

Chapter # 1: What Is CrossFit?

You have probably been hearing about this word and how it is magically transforming ordinary people into strength machines, with great looking bodies. And without question, CrossFit is almost all the things people say it is.

The definition says it is a strength and conditioning program aimed at building a strong and balanced body. But, what distinguishes it from other programs is that the workouts are constantly varied. It is unlikely for one to have a single exercise more than once in the same week.

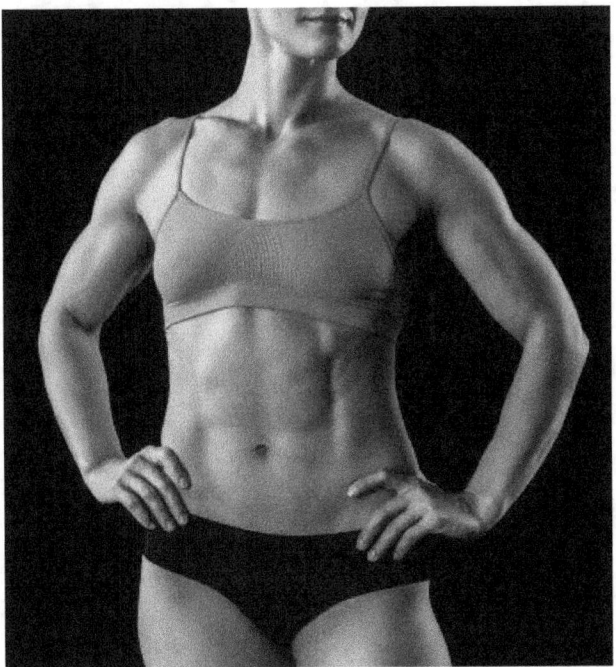

Nearly all aspects of CrossFit are borrowed from weight lifting, cardio, core training, and a few more. In the end, you really get a body capable of doing just about any workout.

Making it even more special is that CrossFit is a community. You will meet a lot of people that you learn to call a family. This is what makes CrossFit work, as these friends are always there to offer the much-needed encouragement. Additionally, seeing them succeed is enough to force you to catch up if you are trailing behind.

CrossFit is hard and challenging, however, it can be scaled down to suit an individual's needs. As with every exercise, there is always the potential for injury, but with a skilled trainer, you will learn all the needed basics to reduce the risk. Missing these important techniques will make CrossFit feel like hell.

Chapter # 2: Benefits of CrossFit

CrossFit is based on the notion of being a jack of all trades. But, as you might know, mastering everything is not easy. Adding to this is that workouts are changed every time. However, you must remember that the aim is to have a well-balanced and strong body. In that regard, CrossFit excels.

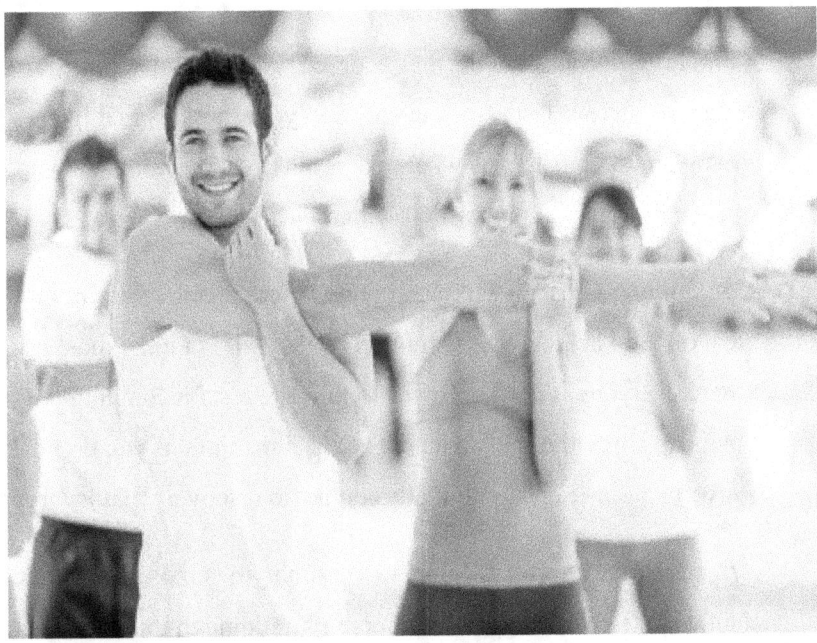

In case you are wondering what the benefits are if you decide to go down this route, this chapter will break it all down for you.

So here are some of the benefits:

- **_Burns More Fat_**: Completing a WOD (Workout of the Day) needs a lot of energy, and it is not surprising to see someone lying on their back after a workout. As you might know, losing weight requires that you use more calories than you consume – CrossFit is among the best ways to use a lot of calories in a short time.

- **No Focus on Specific Muscles**: With traditional exercises, you will either be targeting biceps, triceps, etc., but this is not the case with CrossFit. The idea is to build a body capable of successfully finishing a 5K run today, lifting heavy weights tomorrow, etc. Like said above - a jack-of-all-trades. CrossFit does not make bodybuilders, rather, it makes athletes.

- **Competition**: Since results are recorded, you are motivated each time to beat your last effort, even when your muscles feel like giving up on you. This is what gets results. There are others who engage in friendly competition with their friends.

- **Community**: CrossFit is a community where members encourage each other to achieve their strength goals. This is unlike most gyms where everyone is on their own. Joining a CrossFit community opens up a world of new friends. Most of the time, if you do not show up, your friends will make contact to discover what is wrong.

- **Affordability**: Overall, joining a CrossFit gym is more affordable than most traditional gym memberships. Adding to this is that most of the equipment used is not all that inexpensive. If you want, you can even join a free online community and buy your own gear.

- **Builds Confidence**: There is nothing that builds confidence faster than competing in, and winning, challenges! With CrossFit, challenges are one thing you will learn to live with. You never know what to expect every day in the WOD. And despite that, there is always that feeling of wanting to do better than last time.

- **Increased Energy**: Because of the intensity associated with

CrossFit, you will be stronger than you have ever been. This increased energy level will translate into every aspect of your life.

- **_Stress Reduction_**: As with any good exercise, CrossFit does play a big role in reducing stress levels.

Chapter # 3: Dangers of CrossFit

As with everything in life, there is always a negative side, and CrossFit is no exception. However, most of its negatives originate from the fact that people get carried away and throw all caution out of the window. Whether it is the thought of making gains overnight or something else, we see many quitting CrossFit and lamenting about how dangerous it is.

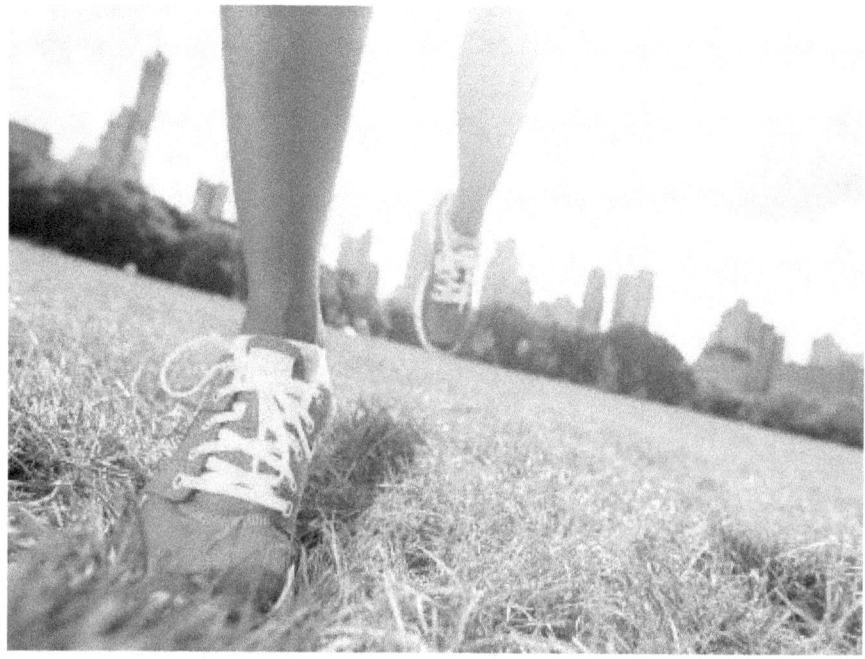

But this is narrow-minded. Focusing only at the two extremes does not help. We should learn to see the gray area in the middle.

So here are some things that are giving CrossFit a bad reputation:

- ***Not Knowing When to Stop***: Surrounded by people you learn to call friends subjects you to peer-pressure. There is nothing more pushing and self-awareness numbing than hearing voices encouraging you to go on, accompanied with the clapping of hands. This pushes people beyond their limits. But, unfortunately, the body can only take so much, no matter how hard you try to push it. If it gives up on you, it does not matter how big your "Never Give Up" attitude is. So make it a point to be aware of your limits. Your body will give you the signs like vomiting and more.

- *Injury*: Almost every exercise you can do puts you at a risk of an injury – this is also true with CrossFit. And now that it has grown in popularity, so has the number of injuries. However, doing too much and not learning proper form of movement are to blame for this.

- *Competition*: While competition is good in encouraging you to go on, it also happens to be a successful way of going beyond your limits.

- *Does Not Improve Individual Skills*: As said before, CrossFit makes you a jack of all trades and a master of none. If you want to be a good runner, then focus on running alone. But if you just want to be everything, then you might want to try CrossFit.

- *Incompetent Trainers*: This is the biggest problem that has affected CrossFit. With only a 2-day seminar, you would be eligible to open your own CrossFit box. Even though CrossFit claims that only those who are competent make it, it is not hard to see that some undeserving individuals also find a way to get a slice of the pie. As expected, these guys will not teach the basics properly or have the skills to guarantee an injury-free workout. So before you join any CrossFit gym, do your research. Only go for those you believe will serve you best.

Chapter # 4: Words to Be Familiar With

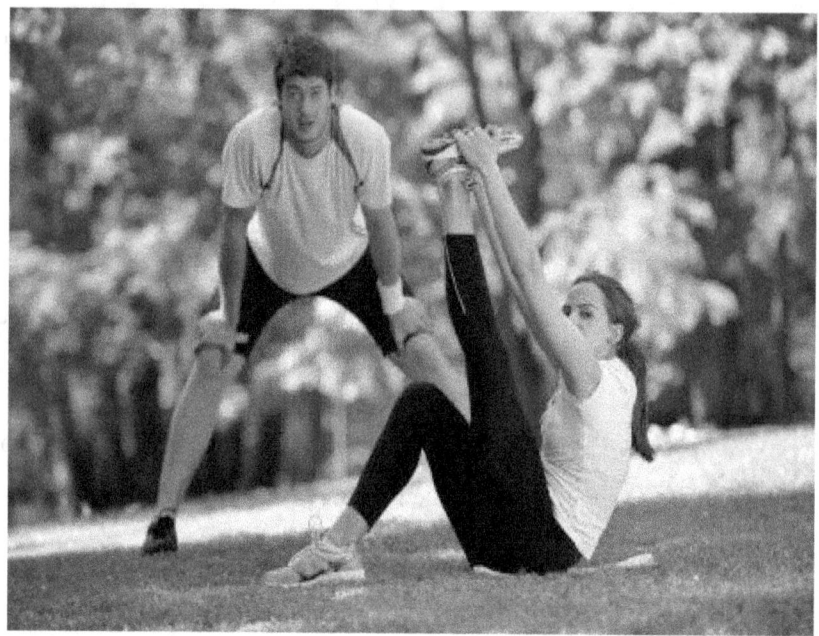

Joining the CrossFit community will open up to a new dictionary of words. At first, these are nothing short of confusing, but as you get to hear them often, you always know what to do without the need to refer to the meaning.

In this chapter, you will discover just a few of the most used words in CrossFit.

- **WOD**: It is the most popular word in CrossFit and it stands for "workout of the day." In essence, this is a set of exercises you have to go through that day. An experienced coach will help scale down the WOD depending on your capabilities.

- **The Box**: You might know it as a gym. But in the CrossFit community, it is referred to as the Box.

- **AMRAP**: It means "as many rounds as possible" or "as many reps as possible." The goal is to do a specific workout as many times as you can in a given time period - The more repetitions, the better.

- **PR**: It stands for Personal Record and not Public Relations as some would think. This is a recording of your scores every time you are in the box. It is used in discovering if you are making any progress.

- **RX**: It is an abbreviation for "as prescribed." Usually, each workout has a recommendation of how it must be done, but since workouts are scaled to meet one's abilities, it means some do not perform the workouts as RX'ed i.e. fewer repetitions or using lighter weights. The goal is to improve till you are able to do each workout as prescribed.

- **BW**: It means body weight and it could refer to such workouts as handstand, push-ups, etc.

- **For Time**: This is for finishing the workout as quickly as you can while following the proper technique.

- **The Girls**: Most of the workouts have girl names, hence being referred to as the Girls. They are a little confusing at first, but once you get used to them, it becomes easy. For example, Angie is made up of 100 pull-ups, 100 push-ups, 100 sit-ups, and 100 squats. As you can see, it is much simpler to say Angie than 100 pull-ups, 100 push-ups, etc.

- **The Heroes**: These are workouts named after fallen soldiers and law enforcement heroes. They are usually more challenging than the girls are.

Getting Started

Chapter # 5: Choosing a CrossFit Gym

So you have made the decision to join a CrossFit gym or box, as it is called. However, the reality is that no two gyms are alike. They might have the same equipment, speak the same language, and make people pass out with the same Girls, but still, there will always be differences.

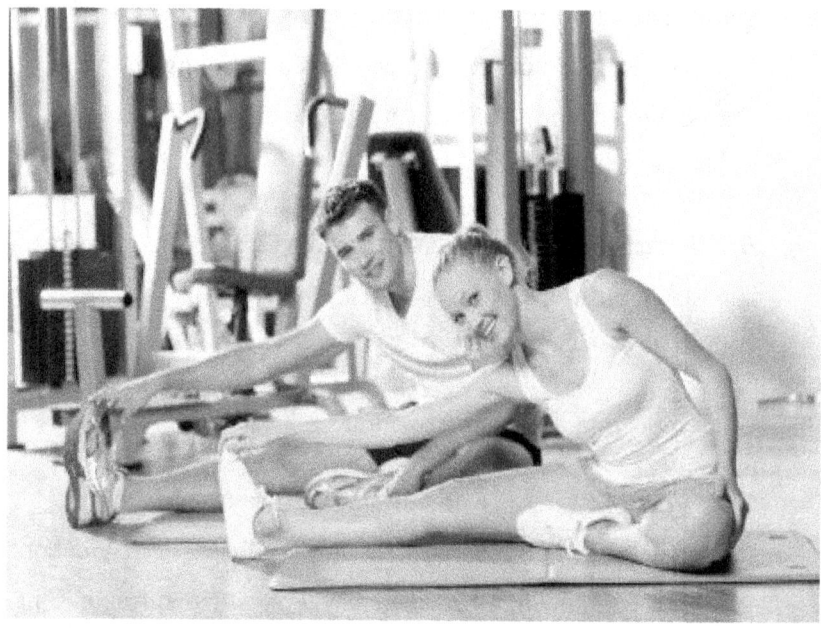

There are now more affiliates of CrossFit than when it was just starting out. However, if truth must be told, not all these are good. To say the least, some are simply a waste of time. So to help you avoid the frustration that comes with choosing the wrong CrossFit gym, this chapter will teach you some things to look into before parting ways with your money.

So here they are:

- ***Cleanliness***: CrossFit is hard - people sweat, bleed, vomit, and do all kinds of things that end up making the gym one of the dirtiest places. So, before you sign up, look at how clean the place is. You could start with the floor, equipment, and bathroom. A gym is where you are supposed to get in shape as opposed to a place where you get sick. So if it is not clean, look elsewhere.

- *Available Equipment*: If you see other athletes waiting for hours on end just to have a short time at the available equipment, then you better try some other place. Additionally, the equipment should be readily accessible by anyone.

- *Recovery*: There is always potential for injury in every exercise. So find out how the gym handles its athletes when injured. Good health should be the priority at all times. You do not want to spend days in bed simply because somebody was so focused on results and not your wellbeing.

- *Focus on Beginners*: Due to lack of experience, there are some gyms that skip the basics. Not only is this bad as it can result in injury, but you also fail to get the most out of CrossFit.

- *Go for Real CrossFit Affiliates*: Simply saying a CrossFit gym does not mean they are a true CrossFit affiliate. So go online and find out if they are being sincere.

- *Background of the Coach*: Coaches are one of the most important elements of every gym. So before joining, take the time to find out how good the coach is, focusing on their experience and qualifications.

- *Focus on Nutrition*: As you might already know, nutrition is an important part of every workout. Make sure the gym takes time to advise its athletes on some healthy diets to follow. Most focus on Paleo.

These are just a few of the things to consider when joining a CrossFit gym. For the best results, try to be as clear as possible of your needs. That will make choosing a gym very easy.

Chapter # 6: CrossFit at Home

For varied reasons, joining a CrossFit gym is not an option for some. If this sounds like you, the good news is that you can do CrossFit at home. However, you will miss some of the benefits exclusive to gym members by following this route.

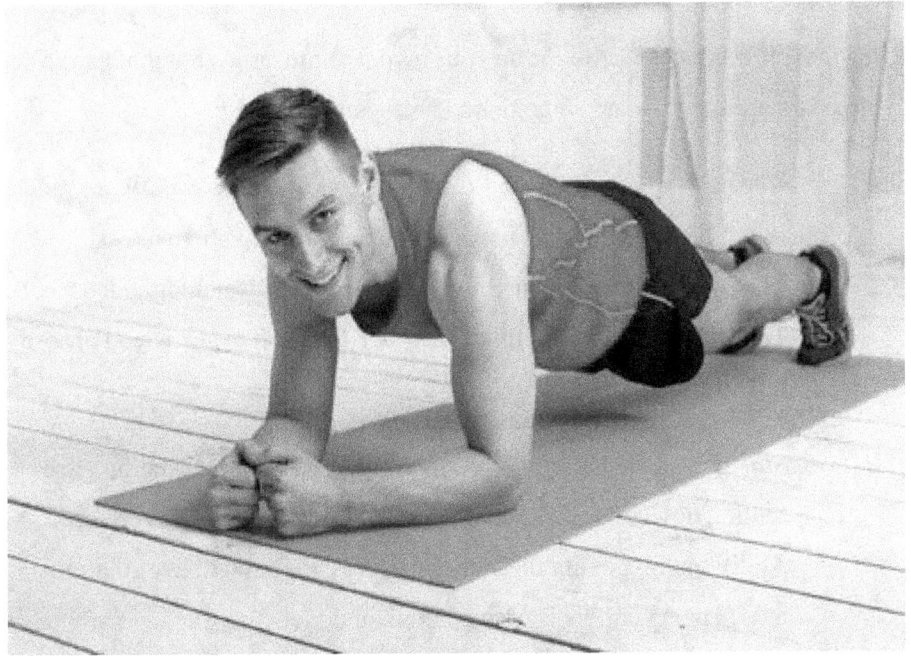

Before we go into the details of what you need to do before you can start doing CrossFit on your own, let's look at some of the disadvantages first.

- *No Trainer*: Having someone to hold you by the hand and show you how it's done is probably the number one reason many sign up with a CrossFit gym. A coach will teach you proper technique, offer advice on nutrition, and more.

- *Community*: Once you know all the basics, the last thing you might want at a CrossFit gym are the people you workout with. Honestly, many find it easy to go an extra mile or do an extra rep when working in a group rather than alone. Additionally, learning with others has shown that it forces people to progress at a faster rate.

- **Equipment**: It is highly unlikely that you will have access to all equipment when doing CrossFit at home. At a gym, however, this is usually not an issue.

If you still need to do CrossFit on your own, the process is not that hard as already stated. Below are some tips to help you do it right:

- **Get As Much Info As You Can**: Since you will be your own trainer, it will be beneficial to know as much as you can about CrossFit. This will involve reading thousands of words, watching videos, etc. Try to think like you will be writing a CrossFit exam as you absorb this information.

- **Start Lighter**: One of the best ways to learn proper technique is by scaling down the workouts to a point where they are easy to do. Additionally, getting the basics perfect early on will avoid injury later. However, this is easier said than done.

- **Find A Partner**: Working with a couple of friends will make up for the missing people you would have found at the gym.

- **Find Equipment**: There is no need to have everything you would find at the gym in your house. Simply owning kettlebells or a pull-up bar could be all you need. You will need to improvise and use what is available. Most of the exercises can be done with your body, so you already have one of the most important assets with you.

- **Stick to Your Schedule**: Motivating yourself to do the exercise daily can be a problem. So find something to inspire you to get your hands dirty every time.

- ***Do Not Forget Nutrition***: Nutrition is key with any workout. So be sure you are well informed about all this.

Mastering CrossFit

Chapter # 7: The CrossFit Diet

Food is the fuel that powers us up to do just about anything. As a matter of fact, our bodies need a lot of it during exercise. Therefore, if you want to be the best CrossFit athlete, you need to be mindful of what you eat.

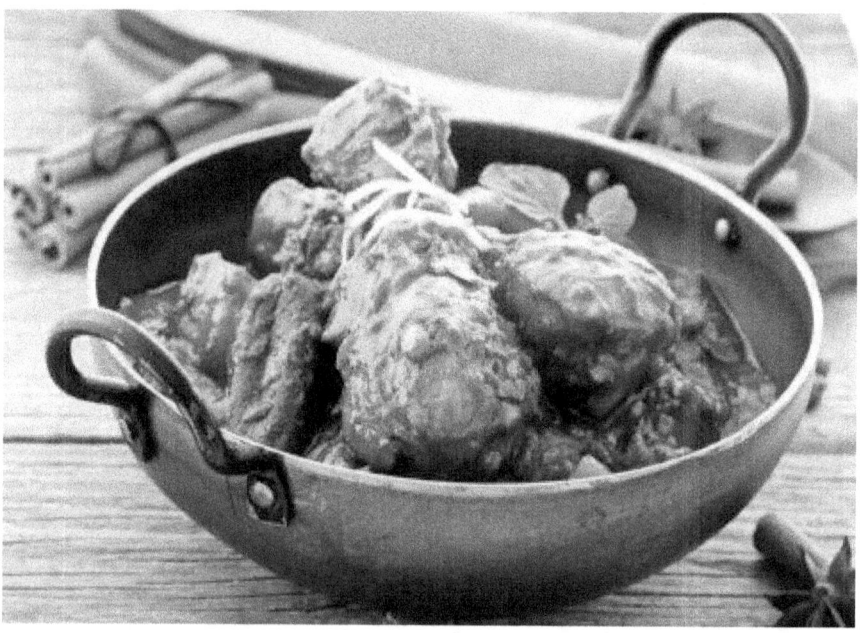

It does not take an expert to realize that much of what we eat these days is junk. And because of this, the majority of us are now sick with diseases like diabetes, cancer, and of course obesity. Theories suggest our bodies are yet to adapt to the type of food we now eat – which is mostly processed.

In light of this, CrossFit recommends a diet believed to suit our bodies. It is mostly based on a Paleo diet.

A Paleo diet is what our ancestors depended on thousands of years ago. Since they had no farms, much of the food we grow today was not present (rice, legumes etc.). Additionally, they had no way of keeping animals so their meat was grass fed. They lived by hunting and searching for food.

The Diet

Following the CrossFit diet might not be easy for many. Without a doubt, some would faint at the sight of food the CrossFit community recommends to its athletes. But with time, anyone can adapt to this and reap the benefits.

Protein: It is recommended that you only eat lean proteins and from varied sources. This should account for about 30% of your calorie intake.

Carbohydrates: All the carbs you are supposed to take should have a low-glycemic index. This means it should not be overly processed and should not contain a lot of unknown ingredients. Carbohydrates should make up 40% of all the calories you consume.

Fats: The truth is that not all fats are bad. As a matter of fact, there are some that are very healthy. The CrossFit diet recommends that you take a lot of mono-saturated fats and these should make about 30% of your calorie intake.

The diet is mostly made up of lean meats, vegetables, fruits, nuts, fish, and seeds. Sugar is strictly forbidden. The same can be said for other foods like:

- milk

- yogurt

- corn

- bread

- beans

- Alcohol

- Etc.

Anything with a lot of ingredients, or that has undergone heavy processing, is avoided. To put it in another way, if our ancestors could never find it during their time, then you are probably better off without it.

Here is a list of food you should be looking forward to having in your kitchen:

Proteins: Eggs, fish, chicken, ground beef, turkey, etc.

Fruits: Apples, limes, lemons, berries, etc.

Vegetables: Tomatoes, onions, carrots, spinach bunch, cauliflower head, fresh parsley, fresh basil, etc.

Fats: Almond butter, grass-fed butter, olive oil, walnuts, macadamia, avocado, etc.

But we should not duck from the fact that following such a diet might mean a lot of changes in your body. There are situations where others have admitted to low energy levels during the first weeks. This period is necessary because your body transitions from predominantly digesting processed food to digesting real food. But once that is over, you will never want to go back to eating junk.

Chapter # 8: CrossFit Rules

Some believe rules are meant to be broken, but at the same time, we have to acknowledge that without them, life would be a mess. The same can be said for CrossFit. Rules help keep order around the community and guarantee that everyone benefits from what CrossFit has to offer.

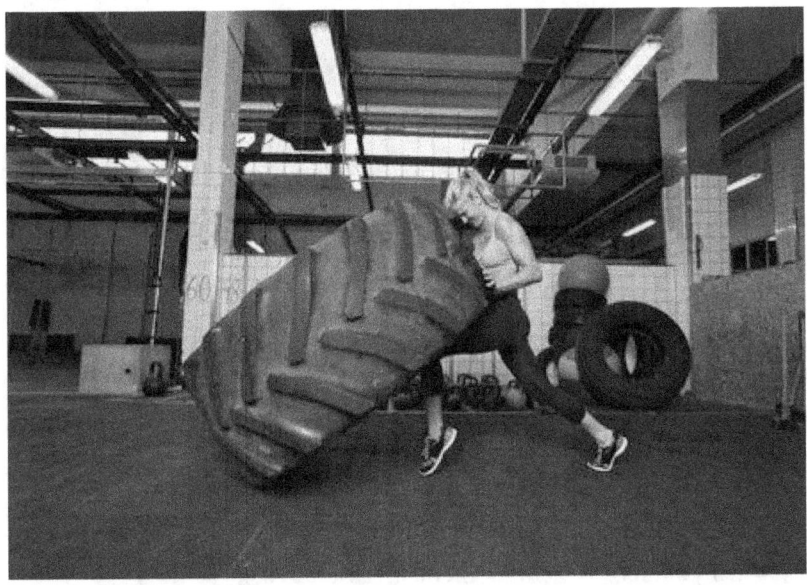

Most of the rules below will apply if you have signed up with a gym. So for the sake of everyone else, try to follow them.

Here they are:

- *Arrive Early*: You should understand that you are not the only one in that gym. There are others who also have paid and want to get their money's worth. No coach likes to stop the session mid-way to attend to late comers. And as warning, some gyms will turn back or give some kind of a punishment to all those who arrive late, so in the end, you will be the biggest loser.

- *Proper Hygiene*: It goes in the same lines that you are not the only one in the gym. Nobody likes to sit next to someone smelling like a broken sewer pipe. So, when going to the gym, always wear clean clothes. You might also consider using a deodorant.

- *Play Safe*: Try to avoid getting in someone else's space. And when using your equipment, exercise caution to avoid hurting others - do not only think about your safety.

- *Be True To Yourself*: If it is too heavy for you, do not be ashamed to scale it down. It does not matter whether you are the only one in the gym taking baby steps, so long as you are pushing yourself to the limits.

- *I Can*: That is what is at the heart of CrossFit – always have an "I can and I will" mentality. If the coaches tell you to take more, they know what they are saying.

- *Ask*: If there is something you do not understand, then you will only kill yourself by being too embarrassed to ask.

- *Listen*: When the coaches are talking, always listen to them. Forget what you watched in some video or read in some CrossFit book. If you did a good job in choosing the right coach, there is no need to question their competence.

- *Sleep*: Every workout needs some rest and CrossFit is no exception. You should normally be getting 6 to 7 hours of sleep daily. You should also remember to have some rest days.

- *Take Care of Equipment*: Despite the fact that it is gym equipment that mostly hurts us (mainly due to improper use), it is also possible for us to hurt the equipment. For example, dropping it like it is some useless piece of junk. Additionally, there is also a risk of damaging the floor if you do this.

- *Slow Down*: Do not rush through the workouts. This is a problem most beginners make. Instead, take it slowly, as you will avoid injury and progress much faster.

- *Do Not Cheat*: You should remember that you are competing with yourself. So if you cheat, you are only holding yourself from becoming a better athlete.

- *Clean Dirt*: Bleeding, spitting, and sweating are all part of the game. But remember to clean this before you go.

- *Stay Home When Sick*: If you are sick, it is better stay at home. Apart from the fact that you can injure yourself or someone, you can easily pass the disease to others.

- *Encourage Others*: Cheer others and encourage them to go on. That is what the CrossFit community is all about.

Chapter # 9: CrossFit Gear

When thinking of CrossFit, many only focus on such things as barbells, pull-up bars, kettle bells, etc., and clothing and other gear are usually left as after-thought. But if you are thinking of getting the best from what CrossFit has to offer, you should spend some time on this topic and be ready to invest.

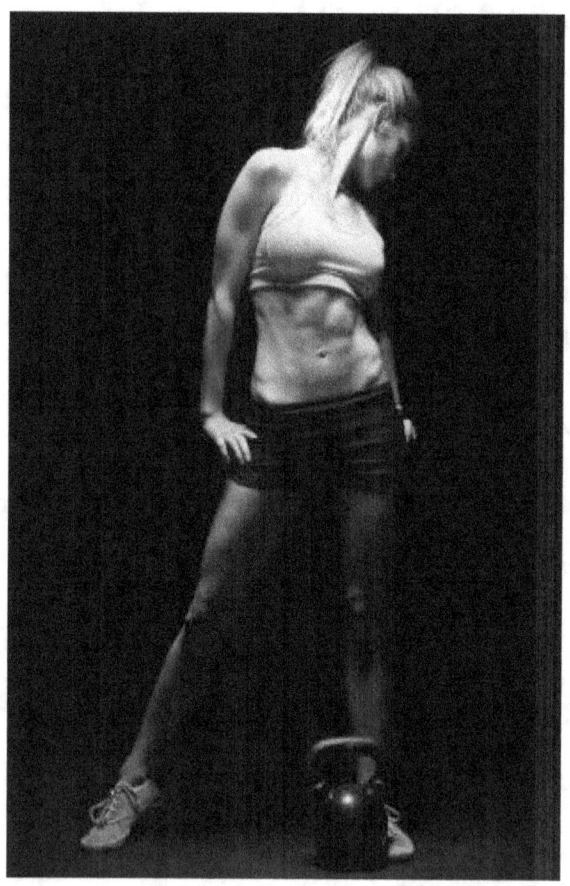

CrossFit is unlike a regular workout - expect to get dirtier than a baby. People sweat to a point where you would think they were standing in the rain. So forget about fashion and only think about function.

Shoes: Many beginners get this wrong, and to some extent, it is understandable. It is not justifiable spending money on a good shoe when you are not sure if CrossFit is for you. But you should always remember that just because it fits and feels okay, does not mean it is the right shoe for CrossFit. An old sneaker or some running shoe might be able to cut it, but it will not provide the best experience. You will need something made for CrossFit. Specifically, you should be looking at shoes like the Reebok Nano, Vans, or Inov8, just to mention a few. The shoe must be flat and have a hard sole.

Shorts/pants: You will be squatting, running, jumping, and more, so you need shorts that do not restrict movement, but at the same time, do not get in the way. CrossFit clothing must be stretchable and not too tight and not too loose. For example, leggings work well for women.

Socks: For the love of your skin, you should seriously consider investing in these. The socks should be knee high. You never know when you might miss a box jump or a deadlift will go wrong. And for those of you who are so much into colors, these come in different patterns, so finding your favorite should not be that hard.

Hand Protection: Investing in some gloves is a good idea. You want strong muscles and a great body, but not rough hands. Workouts like pull-ups, muscles ups, and weightlifting are known to tear hands and leave them feeling like hardwood.

Notebook: Keeping track of your scores is a good way to know if you are making progress. Remember that you are only competing with yourself. So having a notebook to record where you are coming from is a great way of tracking your progress.

Water: No car would run without fuel, and the same concept can be applied to your body and water. So before hitting the gym, make sure you have a good bottle of water. Some gyms will provide this.

Chapter # 10: CrossFit Exercises to Try

Like stated earlier in the book, it is possible to do CrossFit on your own. As a matter of fact, beginners do not necessarily need to sign up with a CrossFit gym. You can get a feel of what CrossFit is all about without spending any money. If you then decide it is something you want to do, you can go look for a gym.

But you should always put safety first, hence the need to spend time learning proper form. Additionally, you should go slowly as rushing things is a good recipe for disaster. But most of all, remember to push yourself as hard as you can. Preferably, try and workout with some friends.

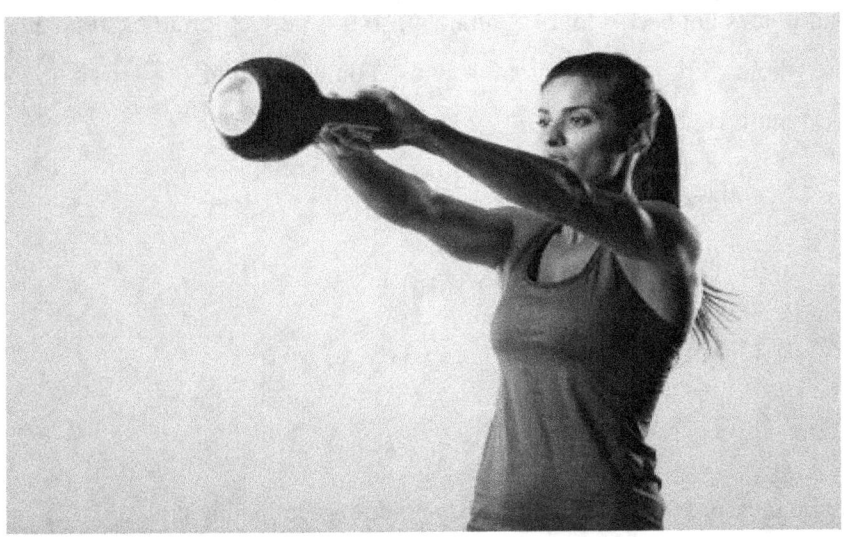

Every time you are done, remember to record your score. It will help you keep track of the progress you are making.

Here are the exercises:

Cindy

It is one of the most popular Girls in CrossFit, but that does not mean it is easy. Actually, it is known for knocking people out every time. This workout is done for 20 minutes with as many rounds as possible. But since this might be the first time, a half Cindy that lasts for 10 minutes might be all you need.

- 5 Pull-ups

- 10 Push-ups

- 15 Air Squats

Helen

Just like with Cindy, Helen is another popular CrossFit workout. Adding to that, it does not need a lot of equipment, so it is perfect for doing at home. The whole workout is done for 3 rounds. You might think it is a walk in the park, but it is not.

- 400-meter run

- 21 American kettlebell swings

- 12 pull ups

Angie

Angie measures the progress you have made since joining CrossFit. It is among the hardest CrossFit benchmark workouts and it is done for time.

- 100 Pull-ups

- 100 Push-ups

- 100 Sit-ups

- 100 Squats

Ryan

This workout was named after a firefighter, Ryan Hommet, who was killed by sniper fire when he stepped out of his truck, while responding to a call. The workout has a total of 5 rounds.

- 7 muscle-ups

- 21 burpees

Grace

It is among the CrossFit benchmark workouts meaning it was made to measure your fitness. Men should use a 135-pound weight while women should go for one weighing 95 pounds. Once you have that, clean and jerk 30 reps for time.

Mary

For even more variety, try doing Mary. It is done for 20 minutes with as many rounds as possible.

- 5 handstand push-ups

- 10 pistols

- 15 pull ups

Chapter # 11: Becoming a CrossFit Trainer

Simply being a CrossFit athlete might not be enough for some. If that sounds like you, then it makes more sense to become a trainer. Additionally, you will be getting some income while doing something you love. To make it even easier for you to get a level 1 certification, you only need two days and $1000. But, that does not mean you should take this lightly. As said earlier in the book, not all trainers are good – you do not want to be among them.

Here are the steps to becoming a better trainer:

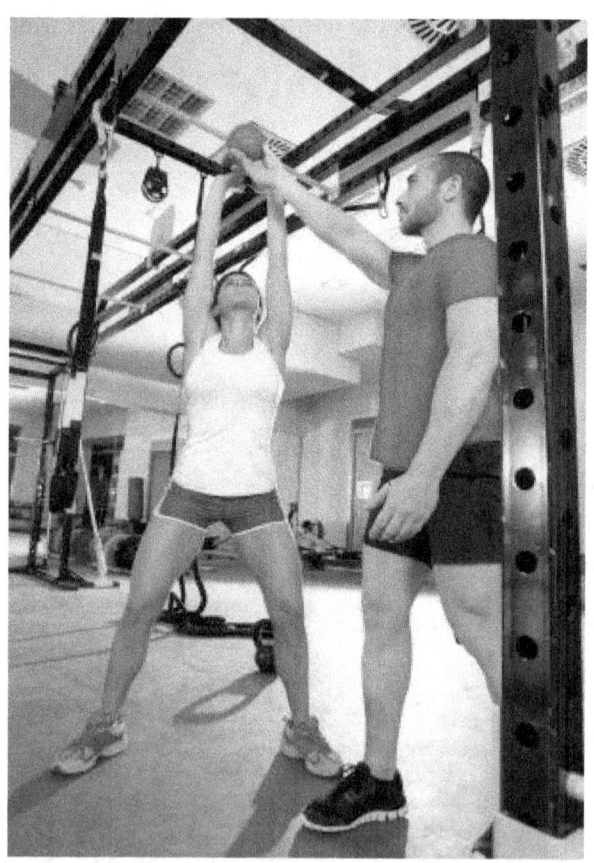

Join a CrossFit Gym

This is not mandatory, but it will help you down the line. You goal is to be a competent trainer. Joining a gym will help you know much more about CrossFit, which includes the exercises, proper form, nutrition, working in groups, etc. You need to be familiar with how it feels to be an athlete before you can become a trainer.

Read

You should be well acquainted with much of what CrossFit is all about. This will involve reading long, and probably boring, texts for months. Additionally, you should spend more time watching videos. You should be a repertoire of knowledge on your own.

Enroll

With months of training and learning, you should be well groomed to finally enroll for a level 1 trainer course. This will teach you how to deal with athletes based on their level of fitness, teach them proper technique, nutrition, and more. If you were sincere with yourself in the learning phase, this will be nothing more than a revision. You can sign up directly from the CrossFit website. The level one certification program is usually done during the weekend and takes only two days.

Use Your New Skills

Once you have your certification, it is time to put your skills to use. Since you might not have a gym of your own at this time, it is recommended that you talk to a local CrossFit affiliate. You can agree on the possibility of teaching there. That will help you gain more experience and become a better trainer.

Keep learning

To truly be the best, never stop learning. You should keep on reading, watching videos, attending seminars, and everything you know might be able to help you.

And as a pro tip, you should avoid the urge to be driven by money or results. Look after your athletes and always make sure that they are in a good health. CrossFit is all about the strenuous workouts, but without athletes, there is no CrossFit, so take care of them.

Conclusion

So there was an introduction to what CrossFit is all about. If you are thinking of becoming a CrossFit athlete, there is no need to wait. It does not matter what your level of fitness is, as anyone can do CrossFit. You just need to have the will to do it. You will lose weight, become strong, and have a great looking body in the process.

Unlike other forms of workouts, which only focus on making you good at one thing, CrossFit tries to make you an all-round athlete. You will be capable of doing just about any workout if you start doing CrossFit.

Practice the exercises in this book, then search out the perfect CrossFit Community for you. Good luck, and stay healthy!

Author Bio

Muhammad Usman is a distinguished medical graduate of Allama Iqbal medical college (AIMC). He is a professional writer who has been in the field for more than 4 years. During this time he has produced 10,000+ articles, blogs and eBooks on various niches related to diseases, health, fitness, nutrition and well-being. He is a regular contributor to several journals related to medicine and surgery. He is the editor of several journals and newspapers.

Check out some of the other JD-Biz Publishing books

Gardening Series on Amazon

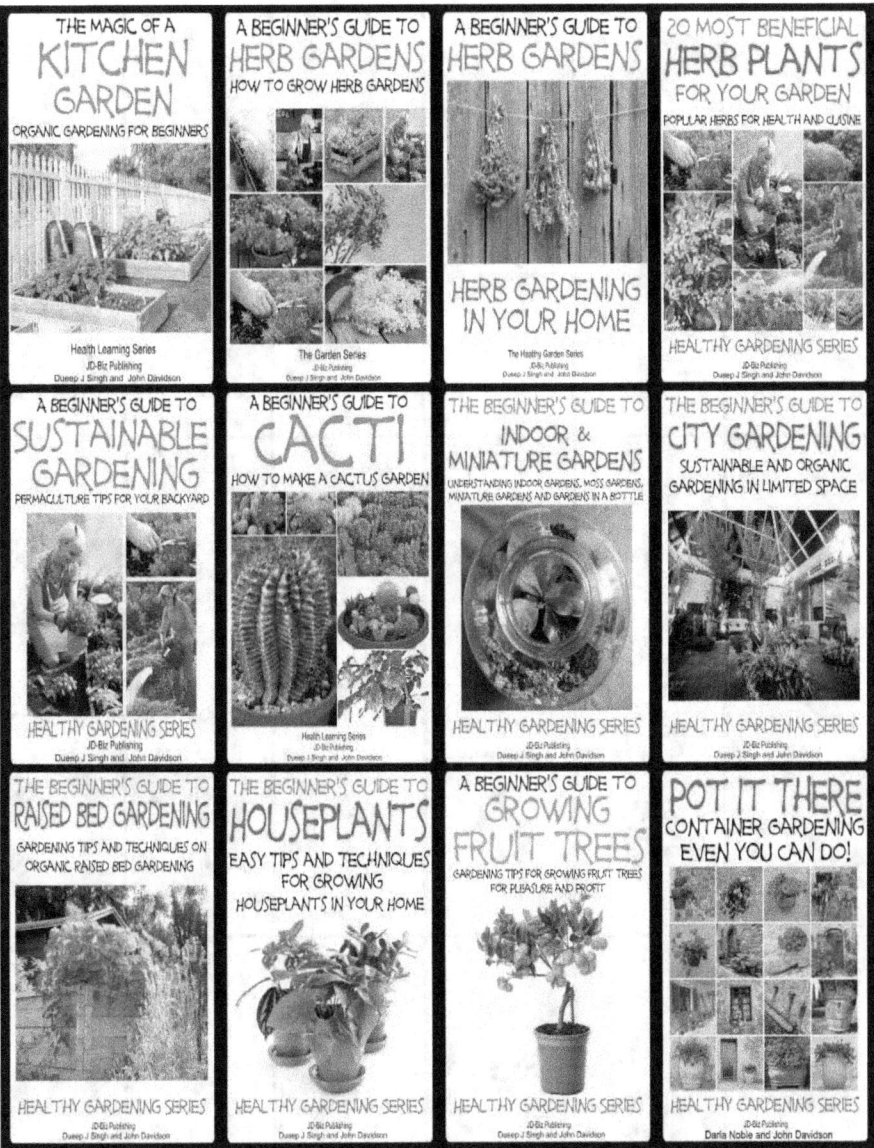

Health Learning Series

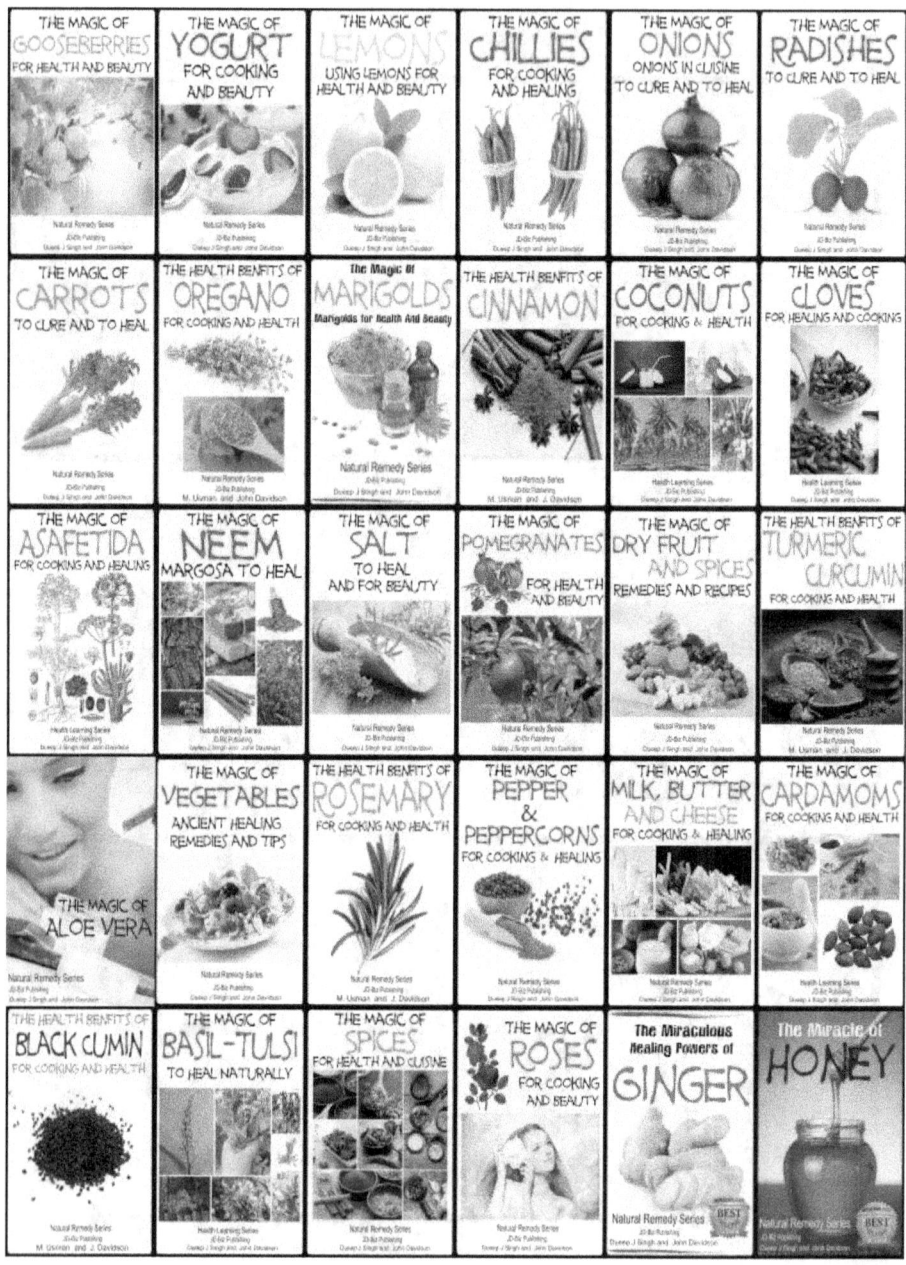

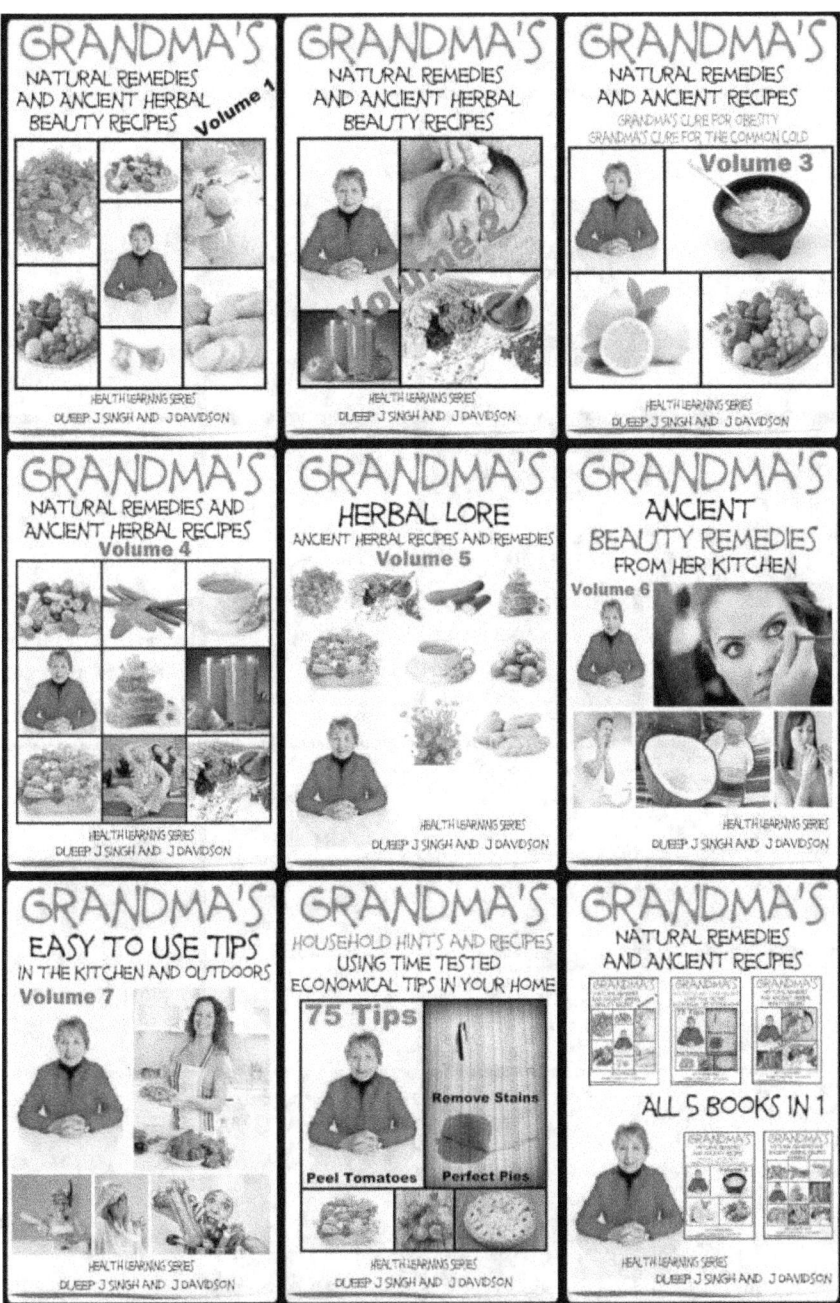

Country Life Books

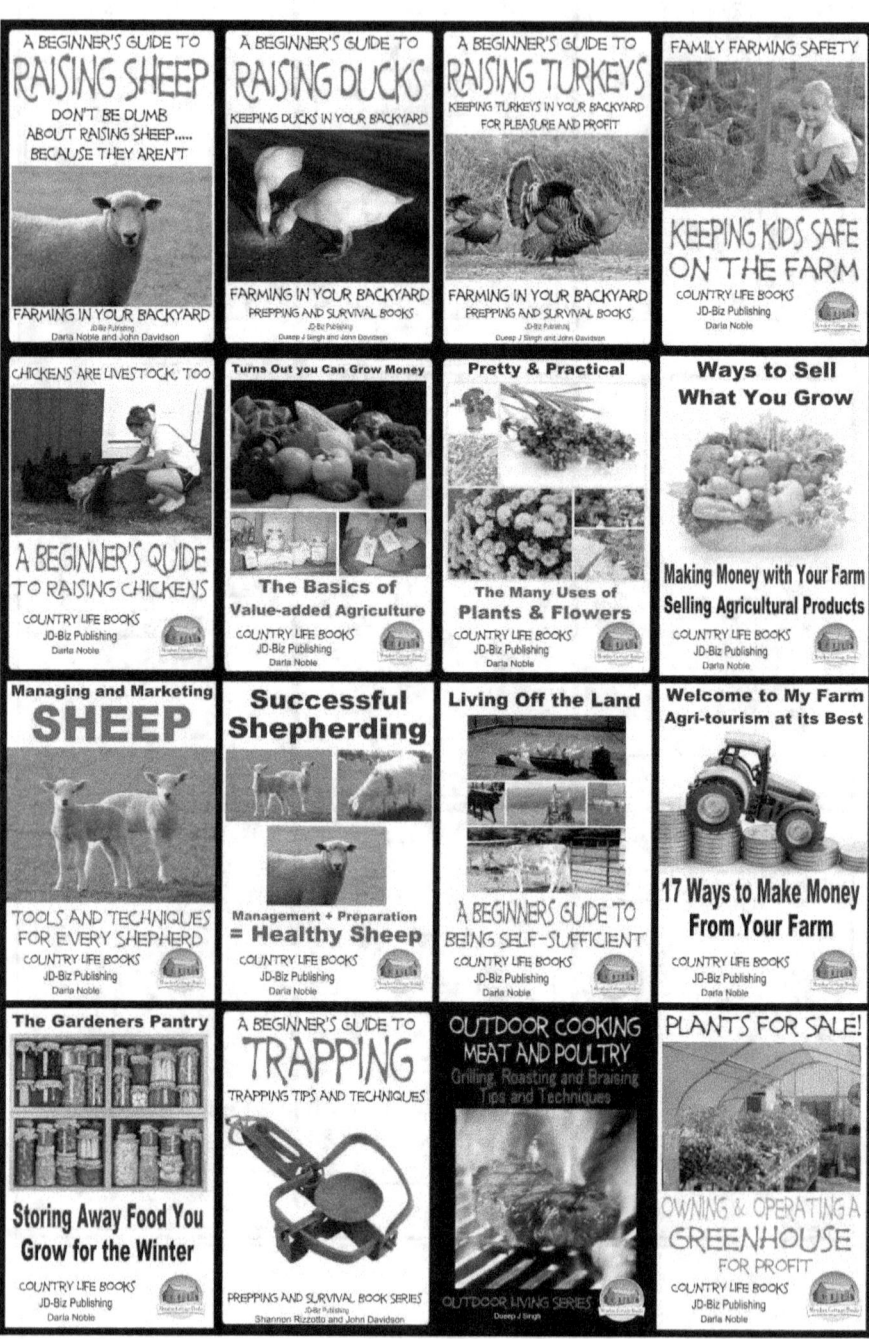

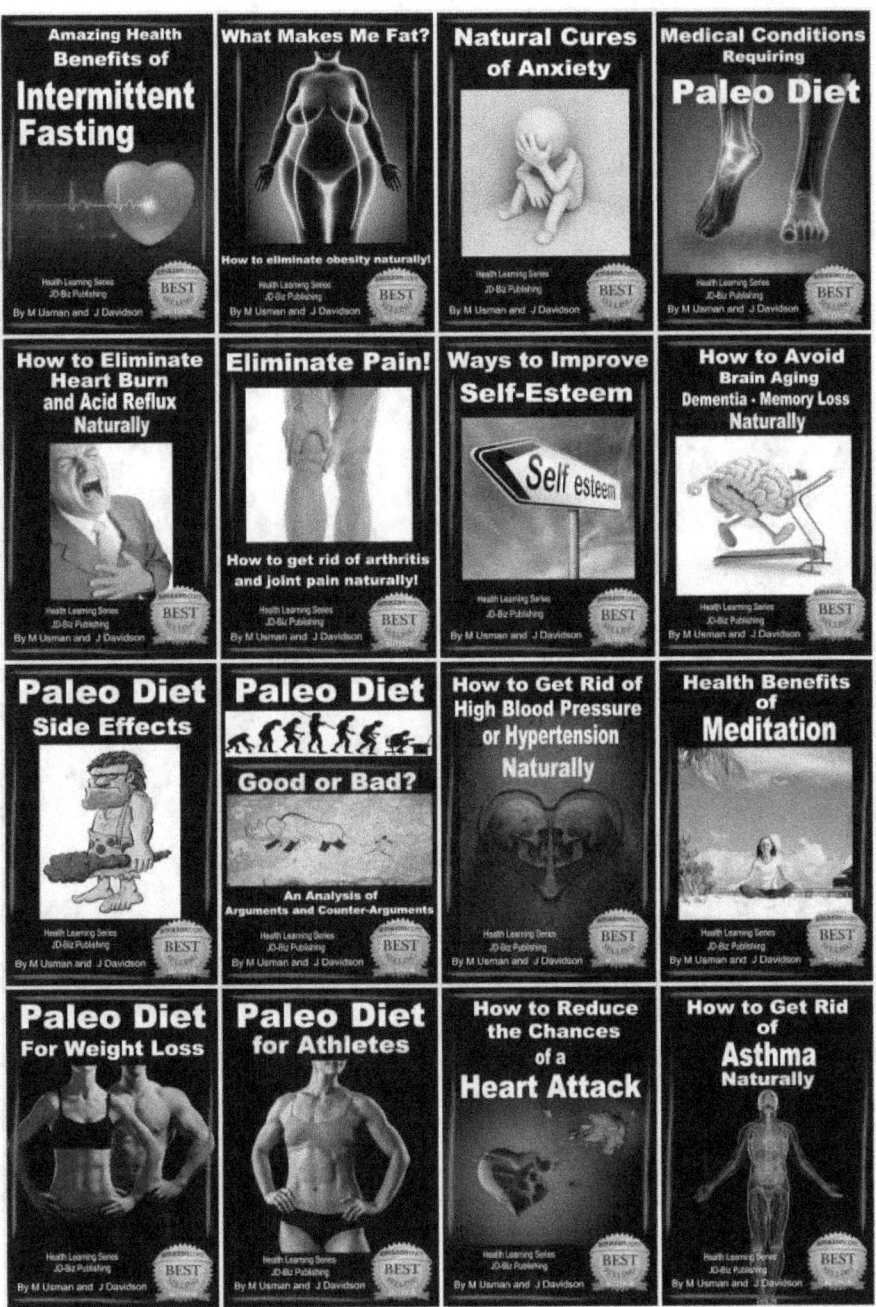

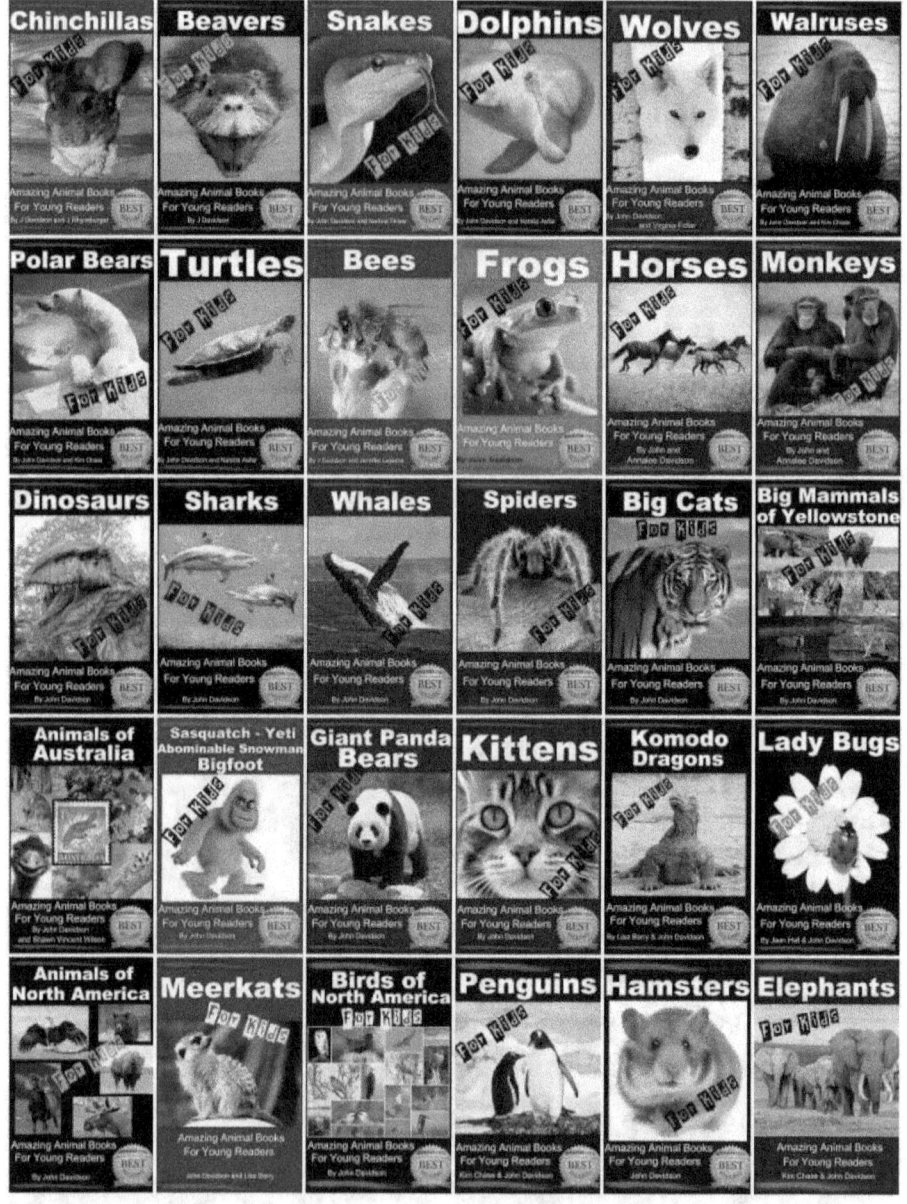

Learn To Draw Series

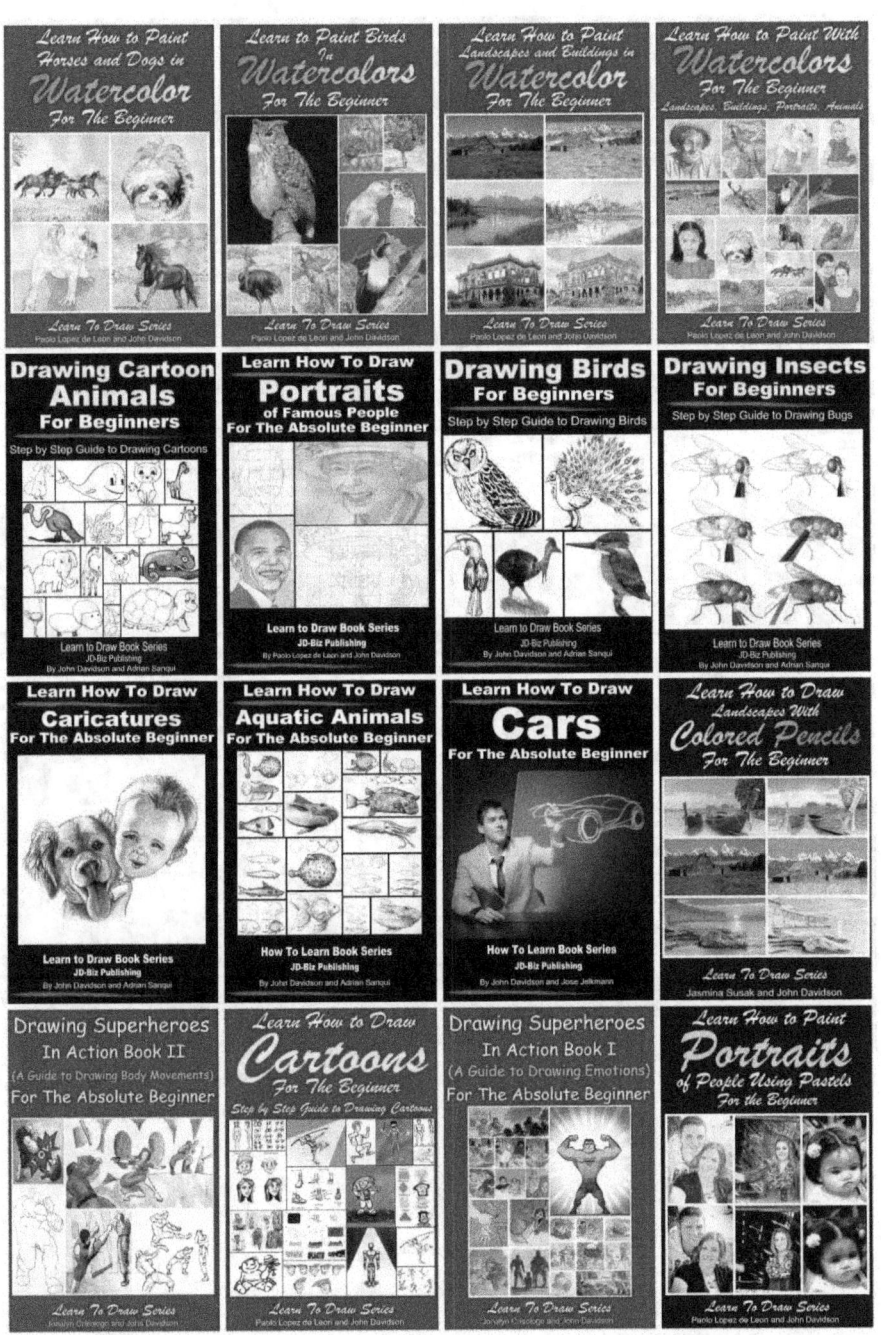

How to Build and Plan Books

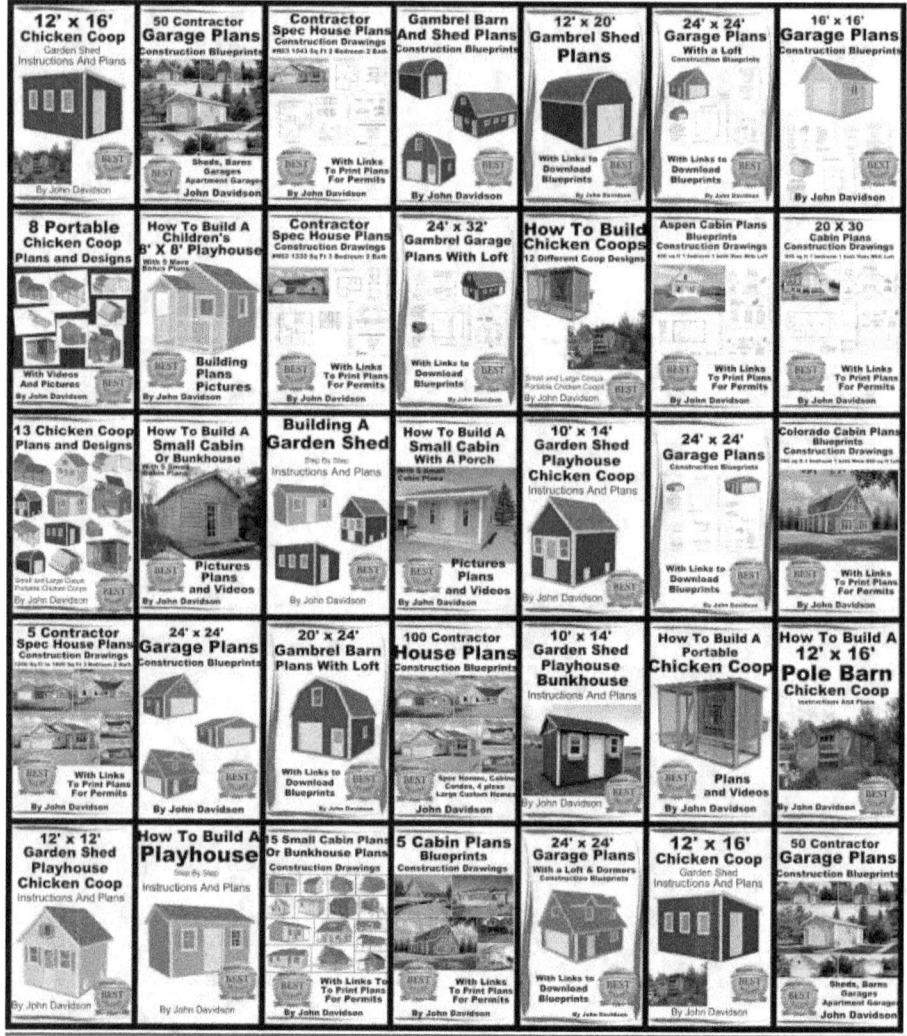

Entrepreneur Book Series

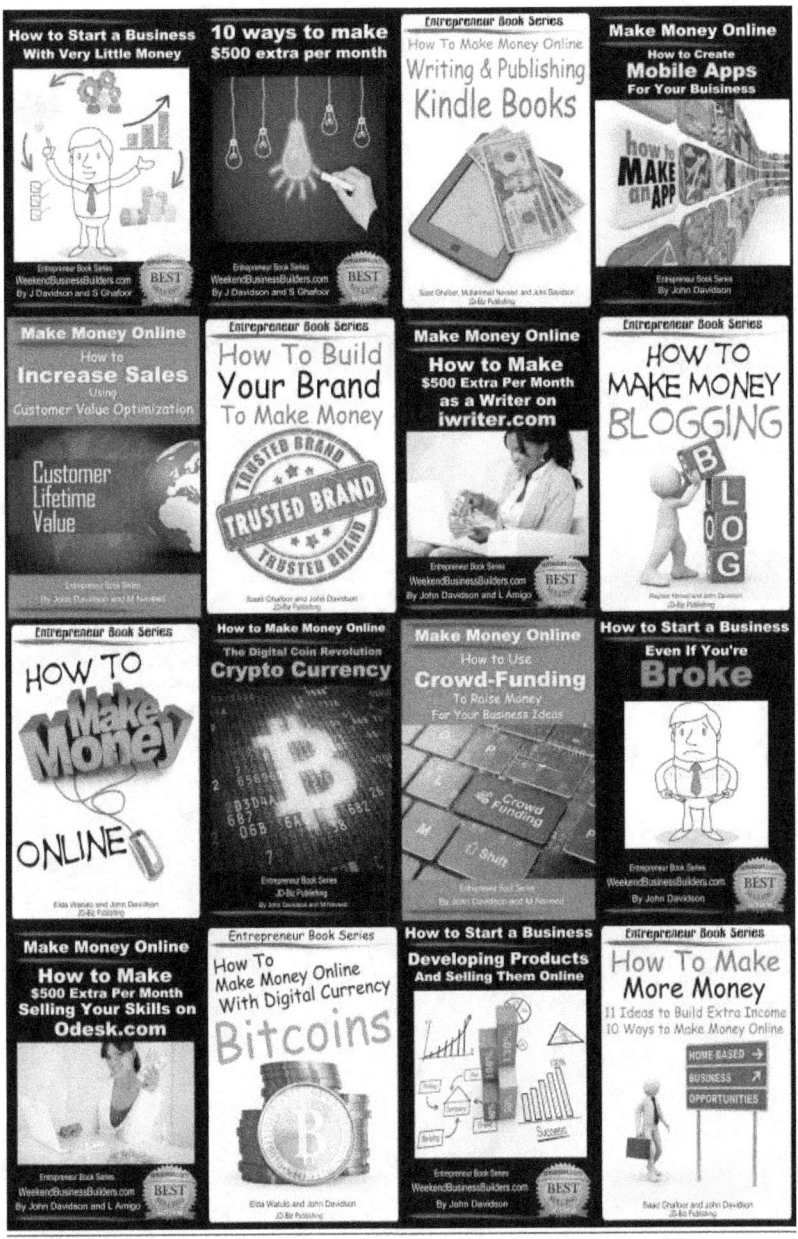

Our books are available at

1. Amazon.com

2. Barnes and Noble

3. Itunes

4. Kobo

5. Smashwords

6. Google Play Books

Publisher

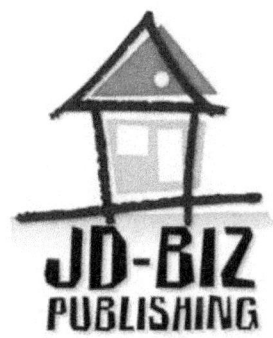

JD-Biz Corp

P O Box 374

Mendon, Utah 84325

http://www.jd-biz.com/

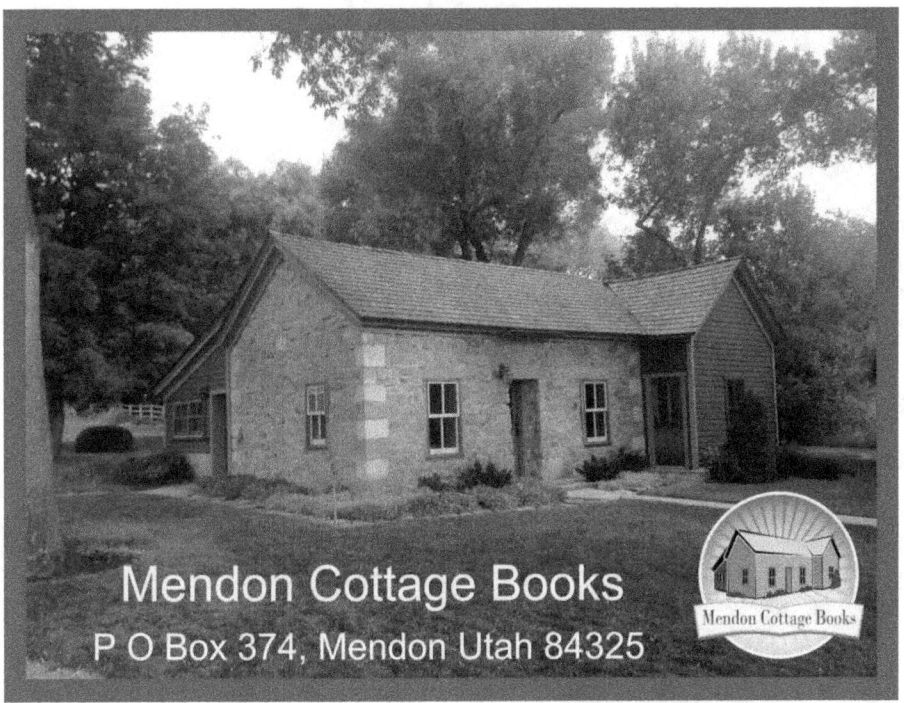